HOW TO **CHANGE YOUR LIFE** IN SIX DAYS

my personal experience

WENDY MARQUENIE

Published by
Hasmark Publishing, judy@hasmarkservices.com

Permission should be addressed in writing to Wendy Marquenie at marqueniew@gmail.com or
6 The Pinnacle, Worongary, Queensland. 4213 Australia

Editor: Sigrid Macdonald
sigridmacdonald@rogers.com

Cover Design: Patti Knoles
patti@virtualgraphicartsdepartment.com

Layout: Anne Karklins
annekarklins@gmail.com

First Edition, 2017

ISBN-13: 978-1-988071-46-6
ISBN-10: 1988071461

Hasmark
PUBLISHING

DEDICATION

I dedicate this book to Bob Proctor and Sandy Gallagher and the programs that they have developed to educate and inspire each and every one of us to draw from within that which is truly inspirational. My book is the realization of an idea and a goal.

ACKNOWLEDGEMENTS

SPECIAL THANKS TO Bob Proctor and Sandy Gallagher and the Proctor Gallagher Institute. Bob and Sandy are truly inspirational and great mentors in the area of personal development.

SPECIAL THANKS TO Peggy McColl for being there to help and guide me through the process of publishing my very first book.

SPECIAL THANKS TO my coach and mentor, Mario Piccone, for his excellent coaching and guidance through the Thinking Into Results Program and The Matrixx Event.

SPECIAL THANKS TO my publisher, Judy O'Beirn & Team from Hasmark Services, for their guidance, advice, and their excellent service.

SPECIAL THANKS TO Patti Knoles, for the creative book cover.

SPECIAL THANKS TO Jenna Martine Photography for my beautiful headshot photos.

When you are surrounded by people with such knowledge and expertise in their respective areas, wonderful things begin to happen.

TABLE OF CONTENTS

THE MATRIXX THROUGH MY EYES

Preface

It was the middle of 2016 when I was feeling a little flat and was very unsure of what I wanted to do for the rest of my life. You see, my health had improved, but I would never go back to my old career, so I was searching for something but not sure exactly what. I had been viewing various YouTube videos on motivation. I had from time to time listened to recordings and rather enjoyed them as they got me excited and all fired up. I was in need of a boost.

I do have a Facebook account but do not log on that often, but this day I was just going through the various stories when I came across this free download of Bob Proctor's book *You Were Born Rich*, so I thought, *Well, it is free. I might as well download it.* You see, I have not been an avid reader. I am more hands on rather than reading how to do something, but since I had listened to Bob Proctor on YouTube before and had enjoyed his style, I started reading the book.

The more I read, the more I became involved. I followed all of the exercises in the book, re-read chapters when Bob said to. I wrote down my list of wants all with amounts besides them as requested I do in the book and wrote my goal on an index card that I had in the office. I followed this book to the letter. Everything Bob told me to do I did.

So when I finished the book but I wanted to learn more, I started to listen to more presentations. I filled in my email address to obtain more information, and guess what? More information followed. The more I read, the more I listened, the more I wanted. I was hungry for more. I sent in my email requesting information at every opportunity. One day, out of the blue, a Proctor Gallagher Consultant, Mario Piccone, made contact with me, and we set up a Skype session.

I originally was interested in the coaching program but was unsure if that was the way to go. Mario asked me a few questions, and I told him that as I am a dance teacher, I love to teach. So we talked about the Thinking Into Results Program, which is a program that I could teach to others and have an income at the same time.

I decided that this was the avenue to take and commenced the program in September of last year. During the first few weeks while searching the Proctor Gallagher website, I noticed that there were a few conferences coming up. Again chatting with Mario, we discussed various options, and it was mentioned that The Matrixx might be a good one to attend even though I would not have finished the Thinking Into Results Program yet.

After further discussions, I decided to attend The Matrixx even though at that point, I did not have a clear picture in my mind of my goal, but I knew The Matrixx Event would certainly help me.

I spent a couple of weeks thinking about what really turned me on. There were only two things in life that I truly enjoyed, and that was dancing and traveling. As I am a dance teacher, I came up with an idea of how to combine the two; that was to have my own website combining a healthy mind with a healthy body by incorporating the Proctor Gallagher Institute programs to improve the mind and a range of dance videos along with nutritional information, which would improve the body. I was excited. I now had a goal. I told Mario of my goal, and we worked on this for the next couple of weeks to prepare me fully for The Matrixx. He wanted me to get the most out of the event and set some tasks for me to complete before leaving for Toronto where The Matrixx conference was to be held.

My bags packed, tickets purchased, my coaching sessions with Mario all completed, and Toronto here I come.

CHAPTER 1

THE FIRST DAY OF THE REST OF YOUR LIFE
WHAT IS YOUR DREAM, YOUR GOAL?

Day 1

We arrived for breakfast at 7:30 this morning, and as it was buffet style, we selected what we wanted and sat down at a table. Gazing toward the opened doorway, people started to make their way into the room looking around to see where to sit and of course what there was to eat. Some people chose their seats first while others went straight to gather their breakfast. I was wondering just how many people were attending this conference as there did seem quite a lot of tables set up in the room. Some people sat down at our table, and we introduced ourselves. We all had lanyards, so our names were quite visible. Conversations started to flow, and everyone was excited not knowing how the days were going to unfold.

After breakfast, we made our way to a room that was outside the main conference room where we were encouraged to wait until starting time.

This lovely chap stood up on a slightly raised platform so he could see all of us, and it was easy for us to see him. His name was Chris, and he was great at engaging the attention of all of us now crowded into one area. He introduced himself, told a few jokes, informed us of the house rules, and we listened intently to every word. Chris explained that when the music starts, the doors would open, and we could enter and find a table to sit down. You could feel a certain buzz around the room. I looked at the closed doors behind us and wondered what was on the other side. What was going to happen in the next few days? My stomach had that nervous butterfly feeling. I looked around at the other participants and thought to myself, *What is their purpose for attending? Is it to fulfill their dreams, aspirations, and goals or maybe just to be inspired and find a new direction in their lives?*

Then all of a sudden, the music commenced, becoming a little louder and a little louder, and the double doors cautiously opened so that no one was knocked by them opening outwards toward us to reveal a large room, a stage, monitors and desks, tables, and chairs. The moment had arrived. Here we go. Jim and I made our way through the doors; there are people lined up at either side of the opened doors, clapping and smiling and welcoming us as we walk in. I am smiling and clapping along with them. I love the music, my body moving in rhythm with the beat. It is very uplifting.

Jim and I make our way to one of the tables and place our things on the back of the chairs. I find myself just looking around taking it all in. So many new faces, so many new friends. While looking around the room, suddenly to the left of me, I notice this demure lady standing there. *Wow*, I thought. That is Sandy, this person that I have been watching at least twice a day now for the past thirteen weeks. My heart races, I say to myself, "I have to go over and introduce myself." I walk over to her, and I immediately notice that she is not much taller than I. I ask her for a hug.

Sandy introduces herself and hugs me back. With a lovely smile, she welcomes me here, but I am in awe. All of a sudden, I am speechless (very unlike me). I smile back and walk away, feeling somewhat embarrassed and a little stupid. *Why didn't you say something? You have a tongue in your head*, that little voice inside my head is saying to me. The next minute, I see Bob standing next to Sandy. *He is a lot taller than her*, I thought to myself, same as Jim and myself. I wonder what he is thinking as he is looking around the room watching all of us making our way to the various tables. The music is loud, and I take the opportunity, grab Jim, and I twirl around under his arm. I cannot help but move to the music.

As all of the tables begin to fill up, I am feeling a certain air of anticipation. Others are just standing there looking around as well, and I thought to myself, *Are their feelings the same as mine? A little bit nervous and so very, very excited. I am finally here*, I thought. *This is it. This is the moment. What will unfold in the next six days?*

My coach, Mario, kept the best secret. Before coming, I kept asking him what The Matrixx was going to be like, and he kept saying back to me – you will love it. Just enjoy the experience.

There are so many different nationalities in the room, and like Jim and me, maybe some have traveled quite a distance to be here. I know Mario kept saying to me to totally open my mind and be ready to take advantage of every opportunity that is here for me.

Jim is here solely to support my goal, which is great, and I think that he is excited to be able to finally see Bob and Sandy in person as he has heard so much about them from me during the past thirteen weeks when I commenced the Thinking Into Results Program.

Suddenly the music softens, and we quietly take our seats. There is a Proctor Gallagher Institute Facilitator at every table with six of us so as to keep us moving in the right direction during the discussion times.

Gina walked onto the stage and spoke to us for a few minutes, welcoming us here and saying that she hoped that we enjoyed next few days. You only get out of it what you put into it, so I was determined not to miss a single thing. *Concentrate, focus, concentrate, focus*, that little voice inside my head was saying. The next minute Bob was introduced to the stage, and we all stood up clapping. When Bob started speaking, we all listened intently to every word. Here is the man who has changed my life in the past few weeks. Because of the Thinking Into Results Program he and Sandy have developed, I have been able to find some direction in my life. The program has given me the right mindset to set a goal and to be in a position to attend this event. For the first time in my life, I can put together the pieces of the puzzle.

From time to time over the years, because of various MLM companies I became involved with, my upline distributors would discuss various aspects of setting goals, getting your mindset right, thinking positively, but they only imparted a small amount of this information, whether they did not know any more information themselves, I do not know, and I was never able to fully understand what they were on about. I did not understand how to think that way. It was like they only had half a story, and I needed the whole story for the puzzle to be complete.

Bob and Sandy have that whole puzzle, and they teach it in a way that all the pieces fall into place, and you can understand exactly what they are teaching and, more importantly, how to take this information and live it so that you can achieve and get the results you want.

Bob was invited onto the stage to open The Matrixx. He also welcomed us here and thanked Gina for all her hard work for this conference to take place.

Bob's first topic for the week was all about attitude.

Earl Nightingale in *Lead the Field Series* talks about attitude and stated that Attitude was the Magic Word – What is attitude? This is the composite of your thoughts, feelings, and actions. Attitude plays an important role in the results we get. We have the ability to alter our lives by altering our attitudes of mind. To succeed, you have to have a great attitude toward everything around you, and in return the world will return to you great results. Controlling the way you think, feel, and act will cause good things to happen in your life. You will become a magnet for all things good in the world. No one can cause you to think something you do not want to think. We have the freedom to think whatever we want to think. Our environment is a mirror of ourselves. We shape our own life.

When Jim and I moved into our house a few years ago now, we decided to build an extension, a granny flat for my elderly parents. My parents are eighty-four and eighty-five years old. I am so grateful that I get to see them every day, and with my daughter living with me still, there are three generations in the one household – I am so very blessed and grateful as not many people get to experience this. My mum and dad have a fantastic attitude about life. They wake up every morning and are always joking and laughing at something. Dad will say something funny, and that sets the mood for the day. They have a great sense of humor. My parents are not rich in the monetary sense, but they are rich in their attitude to life.

How do you wake up each morning?

Have you ever sat down and thought about your attitude?

Attitude is everything, and Earl Nightingale was right in saying that attitude really is "The Magic Word" for creating success in life.

Bob was telling us about his younger life and how he started reading Napoleon Hill's book *Think and Grow Rich* and how his life changed dramatically, increasing his yearly income into a monthly income. Bob was also saying that he really wanted to know why his life had changed so much, so he spent the next few years trying to find out why this had occurred. Bob was committed to following proven direction in Napoleon Hill's book *Think and Grow Rich*. Bob had made a commitment to himself to read this book every day for the rest of his life.

To be successful in life, you also have to be disciplined. Disciplined to do what is required to achieve. I am the only one that can give myself a command and follow it. If you want to improve your results, then you have to discipline yourself and stick to it. There is no use in half-hearted attempts.

Since commencing the Thinking Into Results Program and also listening to various Earl Nightingale recordings, I am more disciplined and organized. I can finish my workload a lot more efficiently than I used to, and I find that I have the time to spend doing something I like to do. It really does work.

Sandy was introduced to us, and as she came up on stage, we gave her a huge round of applause as well. I thought to myself that she was so well-dressed and everything was just perfect, not a hair out of place.

Sandy began by telling us the story of her life and how she became involved with Bob Proctor and, most importantly, the decision she made that changed her life. This story started just the same way as you and me, attending a Bob Proctor Conference, but now Sandy has such a major role in the Proctor Gallagher Institute. Sandy followed her dream, her goal. Sandy made the decision; she was willing and able and had the belief in herself, her goal, and her decision.

Do you have that kind of belief in yourself to make a decision that will change the direction of your life?

Prior to attending The Matrixx, I was developing an idea, a goal that I was working on, but I did not have belief in my abilities to achieve this goal. Listening to Sandy's story was very inspiring. I realized from that moment, I had to start believing in me, believing in my goal, my dream. I noticed that once I made the decision to get what I want, to go after my dream/goal, I fantasized about it more and more. I fell more in love with it. The more I imaged it in my mind, the bigger the pictures developed, and new ideas started to emerge, and the more I loved it.

Remember – "Change is inevitable, personal growth is a choice." It is not who you think you are that is holding you back; it is who you think you're not. If you look into a mirror, what is the kind of image you see of yourself? Is that the image of a person you want to be? If not, you have the ability to change it.

The image I have of myself is controlling what I do. Today, I have learned that I have to change my self-image to change my results.

What a first day. It re-affirmed a lot of topics I had already been studying, and repetition is necessary for learning. It is the repetition on a continuous basis that gets the results we want. I thoroughly enjoyed my day and did not want it to end. My mind was abuzz with thoughts from the day.

I learned that with the right attitude, and once a decision is made to achieve your goal, everything would follow. Having belief and a good self-image in one's being is the key to getting the results you desire.

Our evening is free to do what we want to do. Jim and I catch up with a few people at the restaurant where we ask each other some questions about their reasons for attending The Matrixx and how everyone enjoyed the day. It is wonderful just to sit down and chat with people that we did not know this morning, people who have come from all walks of life and different countries around the world. The strangers' faces we saw this morning at breakfast are now becoming familiar faces. New friendships are forming. We excitedly exchange business cards, and when we finish our evening meal, Jim and I decide to leave the rest of them to enjoy the remainder of their evening.

A very pleasant evening.

"*A great attitude does much more than turn on the lights in our worlds; it seems to magically connect us to all sorts of serendipitous opportunities that were somehow absent before the change.*"

~ Napoleon Hill

CHAPTER 2

AN ATTITUDE OF GRATITUDE

Day 2

A new day has dawned. I looked outside, and it was a beautiful morning. Plenty of blue sky, and as I opened the large sliding door to the balcony, I noticed that the air was a little fresh. There is a certain calmness about early mornings; you have time to think before the rush of the day begins.

After our breakfast, it is time once again to congregate in the hallway outside the venue. Chris is welcoming us, and the mood is very light. Chris is extremely entertaining, and when he starts speaking, everyone immediately finishes their conversations to listen. There is a different vibe today. It is not the nervous anticipation of our first morning. You can feel everyone's excitement starting to grow. The noise level this morning is slightly louder than yesterday. Chris has finished his speech, and we have a few moments to spare before the doors open. I see someone whom I have not met before, so I go over, introduce myself and exchange pleasantries and business cards. *So many people to meet, so little time*, I thought.

The next minute, the music commences, doors open, and the facilitators are once again lined up on either side of the doorway, clapping, smiling, and welcoming us. We give them a high five as we pass each one. Then I meet Brian Proctor. He gave me the warmest welcome and a big hug. What a welcome. I really felt special. For a split second, I felt as if I were the only one there. A few people like me were dancing around. What an exciting way to commence the day.

We have been asked to sit at different tables throughout each day of the conference so that we can get to know as many people as possible and different facilitators as well.

Our first topic today is gratitude. In the book *The Science of Getting Rich*, there is a line that we should remember when something goes a little haywire in our life. The whole process of mental adjustment and attunement can be summed up in one word – Gratitude. What do I mean by this? When we have a situation in our life, e.g., money worries, job loss, etc., we tend to focus on the problem, and when we do that the problem grows. We need to make a mental adjustment to stop focusing on the negative situation and start thinking about what outcome we would like. The second part of that line is about Attunement because getting in tune puts you in harmony with the Law, the source of supply, bringing in more of what you want in your life. When things in life seem to be piling up, sit quietly for a moment, look around you and see all of the wonderful things that you have got, and be grateful for what you have. When you do this, your whole attitude changes immediately. Change the way you look at any problems that arise.

Earl Nightingale once stated:

"Your problem is to bridge the gap which exists between where you are now and the goal you intend to reach."

Further to that, Norman Vincent Peale once said in a lecture to an audience, the more problems you have, the more alive you are. If you do not have any problems, you should get down on your knees and ask the Lord, "What is wrong with me? Don't you trust me anymore? Send me some problems. Because the only people who do not have any problems are in a cemetery."

A good exercise is to have a gratitude diary beside your bed so that when you wake every morning, you can write down what you are grateful for. I like this exercise because it really makes me think of what I have, what I have achieved, what I am about to achieve and all the help I am receiving to accomplish my goal. It also makes me appreciate my life, my family, and my friends. So often, we live day by day from sunrise to sunset without giving it a single thought. It is like we are just living; our movements are routine, just like a robot. This exercise is great for me because I learn to adjust the way I think so that I dismiss all negative thoughts and replace them with only positive ones.

Would you like you if you met you?

What kind of energy are you putting out? Positive or negative?

About a year ago, I read about *The Seven Day Mental Diet: How to Change Your Life in a Week* by Emmet Fox, written in 1935. If you feel that your thoughts need a bit of a positive boost, or you just want to try something different, I certainly would recommend it. You have to only think positive thoughts for seven days in a row, and if you miss a day or have a negative thought, then you have to start over from the beginning.

Well, I made the decision and committed myself to give it a go. The moment any negative thought entered my mind, I consciously dismissed it. I can tell you one thing, I did a lot of talking to myself in those seven days, and I managed to complete the exercise. I must admit, I did feel a whole lot better for it. It certainly changed my way of thinking, and even though I thought it would be extremely difficult, as each day passed, my mind became better tuned in for the positive outlook. Wasn't it Earl Nightingale who said: "Positive thinkers get positive results"?

As we discussed yesterday, we have to have belief in what we are capable of achieving and how to develop mental strength through our mental faculty, WILL, to achieve our goals. This is a marvelous tool to develop. With the power of your will, you can hold one picture on the screen of your mind to the exclusion of all outside distractions. The will gives you the ability to focus, to concentrate on one thing. When you learn to concentrate on one thing, you can concentrate on anything. Your will makes your mind stronger. You use your will to stop all the things coming into your mind from the outside world that you do not like. Your will focuses on the ability to achieve by becoming a master at whatever you do because then there is difficulty in replacing you. This is the basic Law of Compensation. The amount of money you earn will be in exact ratio to:

1. The NEED for what you do

2. The ABILITY to do it

3. The DIFFICULTY in replacing you

Bob said that we could just focus on the second step, and be the best you can be. Become very good at what you do so that it will become very difficult to replace you.

We were all asked to do this exercise. I had to write a letter to myself that I was going to open in one year. Tell myself what I have accomplished and what I am most proud of about myself. I just sat there for a moment, but it felt like ages just staring at my blank page. I glanced around the table, and people were already busily writing. I looked up at the stage and then to the ceiling as if I was trying to ask for divine intervention. What am I going to write? Then all of a sudden, it came to me. What am I here for? What is my goal that I have been working on for the past few weeks? What do I want to achieve? I had to write the letter as if I had already achieved my goals and the kind of life I wanted to be living. I started to write, and I had all this information I wanted to write down as quickly as I could before I forgot it. When everyone in the room had finished, we then placed the letter in an envelope, which will be mailed to us in one year's time. Won't it be interesting to see how far I have come? I feel this will make me accountable. Now that I have written it out to myself, I have to do it. What a great concept. I cannot wait to see how much I accomplish in that time.

"I would maintain that thanks are the highest form of thought, and that gratitude is happiness doubled by wonder."

~ Gilbert K. Chesterton – 1874-1936,
Writer and Theologian

CHAPTER 3

A BUBBLING MELTING POT – THE BIRTH OF IDEAS

Day 3

Here we are again. After a delicious start to the day, we find ourselves waiting in the hallway. The raised level of conversational noise indicates that Bob, Sandy, and the team are certainly working their magic. The room is buzzing. Out of the blue, someone will come up to you and express their new idea and ask for your thoughts and opinions. That immediately draws more people into the conversation, and you have people expressing their thoughts and ideas on various topics. It feels like a very large pot that has been stirred, and all these ideas and thoughts are bubbling over; some are flying out like splashes of hot bubbling liquid wanting to escape. I do not think I have ever been this exhausted and exhilarated at the same time before. You cannot help but get swept up in it.

Jim, who came along to support me, has been thinking a lot about what Sandy and Bob have been teaching us at this conference and has decided that we would like to become T.I.R. (Thinking Into Results) Consultants just like a few others that have just signed up in the last couple of days. He has decided after following a positive thinking lifestyle for the past forty years that he would like to follow in Bob's footsteps and teach this program to others. Jim has now a goal of his own. He told me that he has been imagining and dreaming of himself on stage teaching. He also mentioned that he wanted to take what he has lived all of these years to the next level. That he thought about only driving part-time for the car racing team next year as he was not getting any younger and wanted to change the direction of his life.

"Wonderful," I said. "Go for it, if that is really what you want to do." I think he will be a great coach and mentor as he has lectured me many times during the past eleven years on the powers of positive thinking and how the glass is always half full and not half empty.

Peggy McColl was introduced to the stage. She is a *New York Times* best-selling author of approximately ten books, and she asked people to stand up if they were either in the process of writing a book or thinking about writing a book. Quite a few people stood up. Peggy runs a course teaching people everything they need to know to have their own book published. I remember seeing Peggy before when I listened to the replay of The Paradigm Shift Event a couple of months prior to The Matrix. That got me thinking. Could I write a book? *Should I?* that little voice in my head said. *I have always wanted to.*

You see, we are creative people, and we were put on this earth to create. We are not limited in our abilities. We can achieve whatever we set our minds to achieve. Napoleon Hill once said that: "What the mind of man can conceive and believe, he will achieve."

Only when you make the decision, believe in your ability, be persistent, and have a positive attitude will the results follow.

A wonderful quote by Thomas Jefferson: "Nothing can stop the man with the right mental attitude from achieving his goal; nothing on earth can help the man with the wrong mental attitude."

Bob was telling us about how Andrew Carnegie commissioned Napoleon Hill to study and write about the richest men in the world and how they acquired their wealth. What made them so different from the everyday person? That book was called *Think and Grow Rich*, which Bob said that he had been studying every day for over fifty-five years. It was this book that changed his life. Napoleon Hill made a quick decision to say "yes" to Andrew Carnegie's proposal, even though it would take him many years to complete the book. His studies showed that very successful people develop a knack of making decisions quickly but make changes slowly; they become aware of why they are so effective and why they are good at what they are doing.

Benjamin Franklin once said, "Time is money." Have you ever worked out how much money your time is worth? So when someone asks you for a minute of your time, how much would that be?

After the break, I was so excited about my idea for a book that I jotted down a few points, and I went up to Peggy and asked if I could have $100 of her time. I remembered the earlier lesson on time and money with Bob. I had never really thought of it that way before. My time IS valuable.

So when I said this to Peggy, she thought for just a split second about what I said and laughed. "Sure, no problem" was her reply, and we both smiled. Peggy has been telling us some very funny stories throughout the conference and is extremely witty. She is a great speaker.

After retiring for the evening, my head was full of ideas that were stopping me from falling asleep, so I sat up for a while and wrote a page of my book. Happy now that I managed to write a few things down, I could now rest my mind and body for the next exciting day.

"It is in your moments of decision that your destiny is shaped."

Tony Robbins

CHAPTER 4

HAVING A BIG AND BEAUTIFUL GOAL

Day 4

Chris is waiting for all of us to assemble. He explains what will happen in the next couple of days. These are going to be very special days as this is where you will fully focus on your goal. "Have a great day." Just as he had finished those words, the music commenced, and the doors opened once again.

The facilitators line up again at the entrance, and everyone is clapping and smiling. Jim and I enter and try to find a seat together and, as this was an important day, I wanted for us to remain seated together, but we could not find two seats free at the same table; the thought of being seated at different tables was not sitting well with me. I suddenly had such a sinking feeling. The next moment, one of the attendees offered to give up his seat so we could sit together as there was only one spare seat next to him. A moment of relief came over my entire body, and I was so grateful and thanked him very much. I was feeling a lot happier now.

The past few days have been about how to achieve what we want in life. How to turn the fantasy into theory by using your reasoning ability. The moment I say to myself that I am willing and I am able, this theory then becomes my goal, and the moment I make it happen, my goal turns into fact.

Studying the Thinking Into Results Program, I have learned how to set a goal. You may ask, What is a goal? A goal is something that you want that you have never done before. Something that you have imagined and placed in your mind with pictures. I have my goal written down, and I have a clear picture in my mind. I have belief in my abilities that I will achieve this goal. It is only when my belief (on a deep level) matches my goal that things will attract and it will happen. My body is in a state of vibration, and that action causes a re-action out into the world and what will be returned are the results I want. When you are working toward that goal, you will be working outside your comfort zone because you have never experienced this before. You will come across bumps and hurdles on the way, but work through it. Keep focused on the goal you want to achieve. Have faith that things will come to you when and as you require it. Never lose sight of your goal. Because we think in pictures, use your imagination to visualize your goal and how you want to live your life.

Visualize as if you are living it right this moment. Use your mental faculty, Will, to keep the positive picture in your mind and focused on the objective. We are the only one that can make it happen. Remember that your plans can change but your goal cannot.

This afternoon's session is all about our goals and what we want. One by one, we are listening to each other expressing their goals and list of wants. Our facilitator is helping us to fine tune our goals and to condense them so that we can write them down on a goal card.

Bob was telling us that Napoleon Hill's book *Think and Grow Rich* suggested that he write down his goal on a card and keep it where he could look at it many times during the day. This action of repeating his goal planted it firmly in his conscious mind. When you are continually thinking about it, you then take action and make it happen. Whatever goal you set, make sure that it is big and beautiful.

You know it is so very interesting listening to everyone's goals. Everyone here at this event is here for a reason: to make their goals a reality. And everyone here is willing to help you achieve. As each of us takes a turn to read our goal, the facilitator advises us on the best way to condense and explain our goal so that the person listening can immediately draw a picture in their mind of what we want to achieve.

I think this concept works very well. When you listen to another person reading their goal out loud, we also are able to offer any suggestions or helpful hints if something does not sound as it should. I know when I was reading out my goal, it was suggested that I replace a couple of words with another, which made such a difference to the overall picture I was trying to create. We are all here to help one another. That is what it is all about.

That evening before retiring to bed, I re-read my goal out loud. I am very pleased and happy with how it finally turned out. It was big, and it was beautiful.

"Set a goal to achieve something that is so big, so exhilarating that it excites you and scares you at the same time."

Bob Proctor

CHAPTER 5

THE AWAKENING

Day 5

After breakfast, we assembled in front of the main hall and waited for Chris to welcome us to the brand new day. We were asked to sit at the same table as yesterday with the same facilitator. He explained to us how the day was to unfold as this day was going to be run a little differently from all of the others. "Enjoy the experience," he said.

The music started, doors opened, and we filed into the room. Jim and I located our table and facilitator, and we sat down. The room was electric, and the excitement empowered my thoughts. I was looking around the room, and I could see the different expressions on the faces – everyone looked so excited. I was thinking that the noise from people chatting was so much louder than the other days. This was THE day we had been gearing up for. It was the pinnacle of the conference.

This is where the magic happens…

Experience It   Believe It   Do It   Love It

That Night: I am trying to calm down after the excitement of the afternoon. I have a little voice left, and I am so very happy. I must have the widest smile on my face.

The only words to describe what has just transpired is – absolutely fantastic, what an experience. I have never been involved with anything like this before in my life, and I have been to a few conferences in my day. I have never felt such exhilaration and exhaustion at the same time. Just think there were 108 minds all working as one.

"It doesn't matter where you are, you are nowhere compared to where you can go."

Bob Proctor

CHAPTER 6

GRADUATION DAY

Day 6

Breakfast this morning seems a little quiet as there are not as many people here like there usually are. Yesterday was such a big day, so maybe they are having a sleep in.

For the final time, we gather around in the assembly hall. It is sad that some of us might not be seeing each other again for one reason or another. We will not have the same level of support system when we leave that we have had in the past few days. The realization of going home and working on our goals to make it happen has dawned on us. It is all up to us now.

Chris, for the last time, welcomes us, and as the music commences, we enter the room, find a table and sit down.

We only have a short lesson today. Gina is welcomed onto the stage to discuss our plans for the afternoon. Today is "Graduation Day," and also today we will be visiting Bob's house. As the group is rather a large one, we will be divided into two groups. Gina explains the times that the buses will be leaving for both groups and what time they will be returning. What a perfect way to finish a conference. Gina said that when we return from morning tea, there will be a bag on the seats. A surprise for us and for us not to open until the time is announced.

As we entered the room after morning tea, it was set out differently. No tables, just rows of chairs facing the stage. We sat down, and there were a few announcements and a thank you to all of the Proctor Gallagher Institute staff, Facilitators, Sales Staff, Guest Presenters and Bob and Sandy.

Gina said it was okay to look in our bags. We received a lot of special gifts and also the photo that we had taken with Bob and Sandy.

I could not help but feel a little sad as it was almost over. So many new friendships had been made and to think just six days ago, we were complete strangers from all over the world with a common purpose for attending, all because we all had a dream, a goal to achieve the impossible.

As Jim and I were scheduled in the second departure group, we decided to take the time to sit in the casual dining area in the main lobby and just relax and chat. I felt exhausted. I shed a tear as we were discussing our individual experiences and our plans when we arrived home. I realized at that moment what had transpired over the last few days.

I was about to change the direction of my life. I was about to do something that I never dreamed of doing a couple of months ago. I had direction, and I was about to undertake the biggest challenge in my life. It felt like I was taking home a new baby. You know the feeling when you arrive home for the first time: that secure feeling of knowing that in the hospital a nurse was only a buzz away and now feeling a little insecure as it was up to me. Jim also had a new project as he signed up to become a Thinking Into Results Consultant. He was excited and was already working out plans for when he returned home.

Looking around, I can see a few others also in this area sitting together in small groups, maybe catching up for the last time before heading home. Some were already gathering in the foyer and would be departing very soon on the first bus. As they waited, conversations were flowing, and everyone looked really excited to visit Bob's house.

As Jim and I sat there talking, a few others came over and sat down at various times. Some were having a bite to eat, and others were planning to go shopping as there was a very large shopping center only a couple of minutes away by taxi as those of us in the second group did have a few hours to fill in.

Nearing the time to depart, we freshened up and waited in the foyer until it was our time to board the bus. It was not a long journey, about thirty minutes. The area is populated with tree lined streets, quite picturesque.

Bob and his beautiful wife, Linda, have a lovely home. It is quite deceiving really because from the outside, it does not look very big. But like a Tardis, when you walk in, there are rooms branching off from the entrance hallway, and as you head downstairs, where we hung up our coats, it was quite a large entertainment area. All of the walls are adorned with pictures of celebrities both past and present. I looked around reading all the information under the pictures thinking what a wonderful life Bob has had. I could see Napoleon Hill, Andrew Carnegie, and Sir Edmond Hilary just to name a few. These are very special memories indeed. The library was stacked to the ceiling with books of all different genres. The doorway from the entertainment area had a path leading toward the studio where Bob does a lot of his filming.

As you walk in, you can see a very large monitor just in front of you at head height. There is a desk behind another wall full of books and a few more pictures. This is the place where Bob films many of his segments. I can see Bob and Sandy mingling among all of us. I walked over to Sandy and asked her for a photo, for which she willingly obliged. It was great to see both of them relaxed and enjoying the company; it feels like they are just one of the family and very approachable. I hope they have enjoyed the conference just as much as Jim and I have.

After a few hours, it was time to say goodbye and head back to the hotel. Bob came on board the bus to bid us farewell. I feel very privileged to have had the opportunity of visiting his home.

Very sad to say goodbye.

Arriving back at the hotel, Jim and I started to pack our bags, as we had a very early flight the next morning.

With our bags packed, tickets ready, we headed back home, a little sad but having gained so much.

Reflecting back over the past few days, I came away from this conference with a much clearer picture of the direction I am heading. I have so many friends ready to help me achieve my goal. Remembering what I have learned… to achieve anything in life, you need to have an understanding of the mind. How and what we think will ultimately affect our results. You have to have a great attitude. We have the ability to alter our lives by altering our attitudes of mind. By that I mean, we have the ability to accept negative or positive thoughts. If we accept negative thoughts, our vibrations will be negative, and our results will also be negative. No one can cause you to think something you don't want to think. Your attitude is made up of your thoughts, feelings, and actions and will determine what success we have in life. If you are not happy with the results in your life, then change your attitude to a positive one. Norman Vincent Peale one stated: "Positive thinkers get positive results."

Discipline is the ability to give yourself a command and then follow it with the power of your Will. The Will gives you the ability to focus and concentrate on one thing. When you learn to do that, you will be able to concentrate on anything. Your Will makes your mind stronger and helps develop good habits. To keep my mind and body controlled to achieve my ultimate goals, I need to reject all outside negative influences that will sway me from my path to success.

We have a control mechanism in our mind, and this determines what comes into our life and how well we do things in our life. This is our self-image. We have two images. One we project to the world, by the way we walk, talk, dress, etc. The other one is the picture we hold inside. The picture we hold on the inside shows on the outside, and if you have a negative image of yourself, your results are going to be a reflection of it.

Your results are always a reflection of what's going on inside. Our life operates by images. This is where we put our mind to work. We consciously and deliberately choose the kind of person we want to be. We have this ability to change the image we have of ourselves and create this wonderful life we want. Learn to love yourself. Be good to yourself. Get in touch with you. There is something wonderful about you. See it – it is your self-image.

The dictionary definition of gratitude – **means** thanks and appreciation. Gratitude rhymes with "attitude," which **means** "thankful, pleasing." When you feel **gratitude**, you're pleased by what someone did for you and also pleased by the results. We have to try and live life with an attitude of gratitude and to get rid of all negative thoughts that are entering our mind from the influences of the outside world. It is important to be aware of what we are thinking about because we become what we think about all day long. Earl Nightingale said in his book *30 Days of Gratitude*, "To be able to live the life of Gratitude, the seeds of your mind must be sown from a place of gratitude and love, not fear or lack."

Keep a gratitude diary. When you first wake up in the morning, write down at least ten things every day that you are grateful for.

Our mind is such an important tool. It has the ability to control every-thing in our life. The secret for us is to learn how to control the power of our mind and use this power to paint a picture of our desires, dreams, and goals. It can also paint a perfect picture of you. I have to learn to control my mind in a way that the perfect picture of my life stays there in my mind and is not destroyed by negative thoughts. I alone have the ability to change the way I think and act to achieve the results in my life.

During the past six days, I have witnessed the transformation of people. Some people arrived without any preconceived ideas of what they wanted to do but were seeking change in their lives. Others like me already had a goal and were seeking knowledge about how to transform the goal into fact.

Extraordinary ideas from ordinary people wanting to change their world one thought, one action, and one day at a time. You have to believe in yourself and your ability to achieve as we all have the ability to nurture our dreams, goals, and aspirations. Make a difference not only for yourself but for the next generation.

Transform your life; bring out the creative power you have within you. You are the most magnificent expressions of life.

Come and experience a truly extraordinary event called The Matrixx.

"Enjoy Life with us, because life is phenomenal!

It's a Magnificent Trip!"

Bob Proctor – *The Secret*

TESTIMONIALS

MY MATRIXX EXPERIENCE

By Peggy McColl

Almost four decades ago, I began my journey into the study of personal development. The speaker who opened my consciousness to unlimited possibilities is Bob Proctor. Bob has been delivering programs now for more than fifty years, and he truly is the best in the business, and I am grateful to have met him, studied with him, be mentored by him and call him a cherished friend.

When I met Bob Proctor, I was messed up emotionally. I attended an event of Bob Proctor's at the young age of nineteen years when Bob Proctor quoted Vernon Howard and said: "You cannot escape from a prison unless you know you are in one." I was in an emotional prison of my making. I didn't realize that I had the key to set myself free and to unlock my potential. I started to study Bob Proctor close to forty years ago, and I never looked back.

If Bob Proctor offered a program, I signed up. I registered for every program Bob Proctor offered and, to this day, still do.

I have attended several of Bob's Matrixx programs as an expert and a contributing speaker. This event has the potential to change people's lives if they are committed to doing so. This is one of the most in-depth and personal programs offered by Proctor Gallagher Institute. The people who attend this event are committed to success and ready for change.

There is a great quote by Napoleon Hill that I have heard Bob Proctor share with audiences for years. It goes like this: "There is a difference between WISHING for a thing and being READY to receive it. No one is ready for a thing until he believes he can acquire it. The state of mind must be BELIEF, not mere hope or wish. Open-mindedness is essential for belief."

The people who attend The Matrixx program are usually ready for a change, and their minds are open. If not, they will have one heck of a time experiencing any kind of positive change. However, being ready is the state essential for getting the most out of The Matrixx and out of life, for that matter.

Open your mind and be ready to experience positive change in your life. Study personal development. You are either getting better, or you are getting worse. Nothing stays the same. My recommendation is to get on the side of "better" and stay there. And, when you do, your life will never be the same. My wish for you is abundant success. You certainly deserve it.

Praise for
HOW TO CHANGE YOUR LIFE
IN SIX DAYS

"I am writing this testimonial as a witness to the growth that has taken place with Wendy over the last few months prior to, during and after The Matrixx.

I had the pleasure to coach Wendy prior to The Matrixx with the purpose of getting her ready to be able to not only attend The Matrixx for the experience but to truly benefit from the event and come out with a clear picture and focus on what she needed to do post-Matrixx. We worked on her attitude and focus prior to The Matrixx and there was such a dramatic change to her which clearly allowed her to take things to the next level while at The Matrixx. Wendy is very focused and driven to create the success she expects and deserves!

Well done, Wendy."

– **Mario Piccone**, Coaching & Training Coordinator
mpiccone@proctorgallagher.com, Proctor Gallagher Institute

"There is no better exercise for the heart than reaching down to lift someone up. The opportunity to be a facilitator at Matrixx was such a gift! Listening and helping to shape everyone's unique and diverse dreams and goals. Helping them break through fear or limiting beliefs and uplifting their self-image. Throughout the six days, I loved the opportunity to be a leader, to inspire and clarify concepts with individuals and then watch them open up into their childlike imagination and really discover what they want to be, do, have and give in this world. One of the most powerful exercises for me was when we wrote a letter to ourselves 1 year from now congratulating ourselves on all our successes. This created a breakthrough for me as much as it was for the guests and I am so grateful to be in the amazing energy of this event!

Matrixx truly is a life changing experience as a guest or a facilitator. I will be back facilitating again!"

– **Nicole Kernohan**, Thinking Into Results Consultant,
Matrixx Facilitator

"My first day…was Wow!!!! Ready to learn from everyone in the room, with all the different countries and people was so amazing to hear their goals, dreams, and visions. Then there were people who were hurting so deeply just looking for a new way to run from the dysfunctional life back home. I honestly did not know what to expect from Bob and Sandy but I was excited to just be in a room of high energy individuals with positive vibrations from all over the world. It was an experience to learn from everyone including Bob and Sandy. By the 6th day, I was totally exhausted with dealing with my own negative paradigms putting me in a box. On the last day, I felt I was stripped down from the inside out standing naked and not knowing what the future was going to bring. I just knew what was taking place on a spiritual level needed to change. If only I could bring the High Energy Vibration home with me."

– **Angelina Liner**, R&L Fleet Management Inc. www.gpstrackingky.com

"I've known Wendy for ooh three years now and it's been an absolute pleasure watching her journey. She's experienced many hurdles, obstacles and frustrations long before we met and still does, yet she persists and strives always to give "her all." I've had the chance to study alongside Wendy as we've completed various personal development courses and looked into one or two opportunities. Wendy has incredible tenacity, focus and ambition. She's a pocket rocket who's fun and inspiring.

I loved hearing all about "How to Change Your Life in Six Days" (The Matrixx). It's obviously hit a chord and proved to be pivotal in her writing this book. Her day by day description brings to life her recollections of the atmosphere, feelings and emotions of such a wonderful event. It sounds truly inspiring. Until I too can participate in The Matrixx, I'm grateful for the images and memories shared. And who wouldn't want to know How to Change Your Life in Six Days!!"

– **Sue Johnston**, Dip Coun., suejenterprises@gmail.com

"Come with me, and you'll be in a world of pure imagination" This is what Matrixx is, and I can identify with Sandy Gallagher when she says, referring to her first seminar with Bob, that it felt like Bob took her head off and shook it around and put it back on, and I have continued to rearrange and reorganize my thoughts ever since. It was an intense six days, which I expected, but what I didn't expect is how close you can get to those you meet on your journey during that short time. They become like family, but I suppose that is to be expected when you share your deepest dreams and ambitions with people you have only just met. Does that scare you? Well, if it does, that's a good thing, and if the idea of getting everything you've ever dreamed of excites you, you're on the right track. Every decision we face is riddled with emotions and beliefs. Quiet your mind, and ask yourself this question: What is your ideal, or as Peggy McColl often says, "What would you love?" If it is to make a quantum leap, if it's to move past your limits, then as a graduate of Matrixx, I will tell you the experience is worth ten times what the cost is, and of course, it would be, as Bob follows the Law of Receiving. The experience of Matrixx brings you back to the mindset of a child, for a child when imagining, puts no bars, and no chains on his/her imagination. They have no "reason" to "be afraid," and the truth is, neither do we. In so far as we know, we get one life here on this earth; it's time to make it count.

Before Matrixx, I was searching, and I suppose what that Galilean carpenter said so long ago was true, "Ask, and it shall be given you; seek, and ye shall find; knock, and it shall be opened unto you." I had always thought that if I gathered enough "knowledge," I would know "enough" to change my life. This couldn't be further from the truth. That is a faulty belief, and as Wallace Wattles says in The Science of Getting Rich, *"people don't get rich doing certain things, they get rich by doing things in a certain way." I had studied Bob's material for a while, but I could never push myself past where I was. Ironically, that was my problem all along. I was "pushing" through life, which, as Bob teaches, "Force negates. You must let is happen," and once I got out of my own "rational" way of thinking of where would the money come from to pay for Matrixx, I knocked, and the door was opened. I made a "decision," and just as Bob teaches, the money came. I am now an author. My book,* We Think in Secret, *will be launching in short order. I now have multiple sources of income. I now love and am excited about the future. I'm excited about every tomorrow, and with every breath I draw, I am grateful for that idea Bob "decided" to act upon - Matrixx! Most of us are afraid to knock because we don't know what to expect. Don't tip your toe in the water to test the temperature. Just jump in!*

– **Rawlin Vanatta**, Matrixx December 2016
    www.rawlinvanatta.com
    www.wethinkinsecret.com

"Attending The Matrixx Event was a definite turning point in my life to date. Up until about six months ago, I was working full time thinking I made good money, but I also had to be very frugal and ration what I had. I met my fiancé and was introduced into entrepreneurship and was delighted at the idea. When it came time to decide to go to The Matrixx, it was to cost what I perceived to be a lot of money, and I almost backed out. My fiancé knew better and that this investment would pay for itself over time, and it would be worse not to go and not grow, and I agreed.

I remember going to the event not knowing what it was all about, just that I would get to meet Bob Proctor, whom I had been following for about half my life. It was a surreal experience, and the first few days took some settling in. The people were so warm and inviting, and I could not help but feel like I belonged there. I was learning so much information and making so many connections, and each day I could feel my energy rising. It was very powerful. When it came time for me to work on my goals, I hit what's known as a terror barrier. This is when my goals are so scary that it frightens me, and my brain begs me to retreat. But in order to grow, you have to get out of that comfort zone where nothing happens so you can get past the barrier and into freedom. It was a sense of relief when I finally did. I left The Matrixx with a newfound feeling of self-confidence and clarify. And what surprised me the most was that at dinner with Bob the last day, I had the most amazing book idea and took action immediately. At present, my book is written and will be released in a few months. It was the application of all I learned at The Matrixx that made this both possible and a success. In closing, you can't ever go wrong investing in yourself, and it is the only way to learn. It helped me connect with myself and get rid of the paradigms that were holding me back so I can now enjoy the abundance and limitlessness of the universe to which I'm deeply humbled and grateful."

– **Jennie Laurent**, JennieGoGreen@gmail.com, There is a better way.

"How Bob Proctor Taught Me the Most Valuable Lesson!"

"Sometimes we are so ready to move forward — to achieve, create, or make a change in our lives — only to find we continue to stand still. We seem to be doing everything right, but something is holding us back. It was time for me to move forward in my life. During a very difficult four-year divorce, I had been studying with different mentors the universe brought to me, providing the tools to keep the family strong while learning more about myself and what I wanted my life to be. I was so ready to make it all happen, only it wasn't happening and I wanted to know why! Many people come to a point like this, only to become frustrated when old fears take hold. Maybe this change was not meant to happen. The timing isn't right, they reason, or it is better to stay with what they know. They may not be happy, but they pacify themselves by living with what they have come to expect.

Staying with what I knew was not an option. I was the person my children now depended on for love and support, and to lead them forward in the best way possible. Like all my mentors, Bob Proctor appeared seemingly by chance. I was intrigued by his presentation. What he was saying was not new to me, but how he was saying it made me stop and think. This man was sent to give me a good, swift kick in the butt and get me moving. I could feel it. I signed up immediately for his event. One month later I was not only watching a Bob Proctor live event, but getting a chance to meet with him. Was I nervous? Yes! I had learned everything I could about Bob and his teachings. The more I learned, the more I realized the universe was on to something here. As soon as I sat down across from Bob, he asked how I was and I let it pour out of me.

'Bob, I don't know why I can't seem to move forward. I feel like I am so ready, and yet I won't do it. What is going on?' I told him that I was newly divorced; however, I had appealed the support issue — not to gain more money but to change the decision the judge had made that would affect our children's college education.

He asked me more questions about the divorce and then studied me very quietly. Then he said, 'You need to let it go totally.' 'Let go, totally? How? What about the appeal and my kids?' 'Let it go, the whole thing. You don't need this. You have your purpose and you're ready. Let go! Write your book and continue to write. Help people all over the world like you want to. Get started on your life.'

A wave of release went through me. It was really an interesting feeling. I felt the last bit of tension that I was holding onto let go! It felt wonderful and I was excited to start moving forward. Later that night I awoke about 2 a.m. I was arguing with myself. I wanted this freedom, this ability to feel like I could move on, but what about the appeal? What about my children and their future? If I dropped the appeal, it could limit their choices in the future. Back and forth I went, should I or should I not? Needless to say, I didn't sleep much. Finally I decided to listen to myself. When I told myself I was going to drop everything, my stomach tightened. This is my body telling me that I don't agree with this choice. My stomach is my spot. What is yours? When I said I would stay with the appeal, my stomach eased, but I wasn't happy. The idea of dropping the appeal and its possible effect on my children's college choices just filled me with regret. Regret is something I abhor. But I didn't want to let go of this feeling of letting go. I wanted to be totally free to get my life going. How could I let go and not let go? Then I got it. When I entered the appeal I had done what I knew in my heart had to be done, and had prepared and got the ball rolling. Now it was a process. I could let the process go – offer the outcome up to God or the universe. There was nothing more I needed to do. I had done everything. Whether I won or lost was not something I could control at that point. So why let it hold onto me even a little bit? It was time to start my purpose and let it all go! So for the remaining three months, I gave little thought to the outcome. It was out of my hands and no amount of worrying would help. Instead, I started to get my book together. I was loving everything my life was presenting to me. I had no regret. I felt free. Finally and wonderfully free. Three months later the court decided against me. I did not win.

Now I would be lying if I said it didn't matter; of course it did or I wouldn't have pursued it. But it didn't bring me down. It didn't make me feel horrid inside. I know in my heart that we would be fine anyway. I know where I am going and I know I will be able to give my children the best I can give them. Focusing on your desire and definite plan for your future can give rise to nervousness, fear, and doubt. Do not despair. Practice your gratefulness, raise your vibration and thoughts, and focus on your desire or purpose. Let go of the negative emotions; they will not help you make the right choices. No good choice comes from fear or doubt. Focus on what needs your attention in the present and let the rest unfold. You are not a fortune teller, so why spend your time worrying about something you cannot control? Allow me to finish my example. I had lost the appeal and had let go of the loss. I had forgiven myself and anyone else involved in the process and I felt at peace. One month later I receive a call from my ex's family. It was a call to assure me that I need *not worry, for our children would be helped with their college expenses. The whole purpose for my going for the appeal had been for college. Although I had lost through the court, I had won what I wanted for our children in the end. Looking back, I know it was because I had let go of the hurt and harbored no anger or fear. I was at peace and accepting of my ex and his whole family. Because I thought and felt this way, I know it came out in my speech, actions, and feelings every time we met. Feeling my tolerance and acceptance allowed them to also soften toward me. And both of us as parents ultimately want to provide the best we can for our children. Letting go removed the worry, doubt, and fear and allowed the process to bring my purpose or desire back to me. Thank you, Mr. Bob Proctor!"*

– **Alena Chapman**, best-selling author, mentor, and speaker, *Your Guide to Authoritative Control So You Can Be the Master of Your Life and Celebrate the Joy and Abundance You Deserve!*
www.alenachapmanlife.com
www.theprisoneffect.com

ABOUT THE AUTHOR

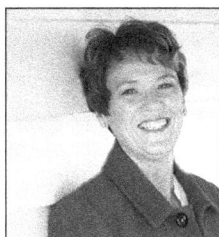

I have always had an interest in dancing, and at an early age, I commenced classes in tap and ballet. Through these years, I gained many accolades and even a scholarship and always found dancing to be lots of fun and quite easy.

Marriage, divorce, motherhood and raising a family bring along its own set of challenges, and the years quickly flew by. I commenced studies in a different form of dance, Latin/Ballroom, and became a qualified professional teacher and adjudicator. During the many years that followed, I enjoyed many additional careers choices, as a travel consultant and in airline customer service and flight attendant roles.

A major life challenge presented itself, and as I worked through the many issues, I found myself looking for my next career move. I was sent a free book, *You Were Born Rich* by Bob Proctor. I was so fascinated by the material in the book that I wanted to learn more. I signed up for the Thinking Into Results Program, had a wonderful coach, Mario Piccone, and attended The Matrixx in Toronto, December 2016. I wrote this book to share my experiences with the world. My website: www.shapeupforsuccess.com is being developed. I enjoy helping people to develop healthy minds through the Proctor Gallagher programs as well as developing healthy bodies through my dance exercise videos and nutritional information.

My journey is just beginning.

The Literary Fairies

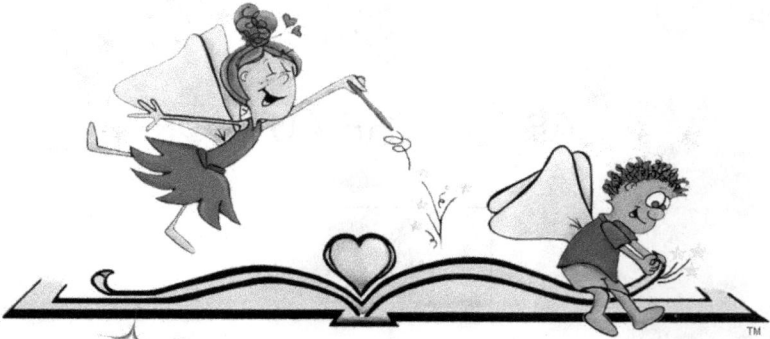

we make your literary wish come true

Wendy Marquenie

has partnered with

The Literary Fairies

who have a mission to give to those who have
experienced an adversity or disability an opportunity
to become a published author while sharing
a story to uplift, inspire and entertain the world.

Visit TLF website to find out how YOU
could become a published author or where
you can help grant a literary wish.

More details provided at
www.theliteraryfairies.com

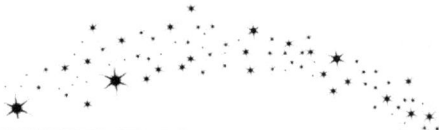

www.ingramcontent.com/pod-product-compliance
Lightning Source LLC
Chambersburg PA
CBHW072017290326
41934CB00009BA/2105